HOW TO DO NATURAL TREATMENTS FOR PSORIASIS

RELIEVE THE PAIN OF YOUR SKIN, YOUR NAILS, YOUR HEAD, YOUR ARMPITS AND YOUR WHOLE BODY OF ALL TYPES OF PSORIASIS

Jessy M. Brown

Table of Contents

Introduction Psoriasis

Psoriasis is a disease suffered by many millions of people worldwide, and several developed countries report incidence rates that are remarkably similar.

For example, in the USA, the reported rate of severe psoriasis ranges from 2% to 3% of the population, while in Australia the disease also affects about 2% of the population.

In addition, some suggest that up to 20% of the U.S. population may have some form of psoriasis, from very mild to severe, and that perhaps as many as 4.5 million people may have severe psoriasis.

In addition, it has been reported that 150,000 new cases of psoriasis are reported each year in the USA alone, so if psoriasis is assumed to be as prevalent in other countries as it is in the USA, it clearly represents a significant problem on a global scale.

For psoriasis sufferers, there is a paradox of "good news and bad news" with which most of these people have already learned to live.

The good news is that, on the one hand, psoriasis is not a life-threatening condition (although it has been suggested that the condition increases the risk of heart attack). However, the fact that psoriasis can bring a great deal of misery to both the sick and their families is not a condition that can be ignored.

In addition, as it can become much more unpleasant and painful, psoriasis is a disease that patients have to treat.

As with any medical condition or ailment, there are many different ways to treat psoriasis. Some are drug-dependent, while others are completely natural. And of course, it almost always follows that treating any medical condition naturally is the best way to do things if such treatments are going to be appropriate and effective.

The purpose of this book is to examine what psoriasis is and what causes it in more detail, before examining the different ways of treating the condition.

Armed with this information, you should be able to consider and decide if using pharmaceutical drugs is a good idea for treating your own psoriasis condition or if using 100% natural methods of treating your condition is a better idea.

> ## *What is psoriasis?*

Psoriasis is an inflammatory skin disease that is not contagious.

There are five different types of psoriasis, the most common of which is plaque psoriasis, which is a form suffered by approximately 80% of psoriasis sufferers. This particular form of psoriasis (also known as "psoriasis vulgaris," which means "common") often appears as raised red spots of skin that are often covered with a silver-white scale.

These skin patches, also known as plaques (hence the name of the condition) or lesions, are most commonly found on the elbows and knees, scalp, or sometimes in the lower back of the person who has them.

That said, they are not limited to these particular areas of the body and can appear anywhere on the head, torso, or extremities.

The other less common types of psoriasis are:

- Gutta psoriasis that is characterized by small red spots on the skin. This particular form of psoriasis most commonly develops in children or adolescents who have a history of strep infections;

- ***Erythrodermic psoriasis*** in which the patient suffers from generalized redness, intense itching and often pain. This is the least common type of psoriasis suffered by between 1% and 2% of people who have psoriasis, which is fortunate, as this particular type of psoriasis can, in the most extreme cases, be life-threatening. This is because in the most severe cases, large sections of skin are shed, meaning that there are areas of exposed and unprotected meat that could be prone to infection (often compared to those with very severe burns);

- ***Inverse psoriasis*** is when the patient is likely to find small red, smooth lesions that form in the skin folds of the body, where warm, moist conditions (such as in the armpits, genital area, etc.) favour the formation of smooth, non-squamous contact plaques, but which nevertheless hurt when touched; and

- ***Pustular psoriasis*** is characterised by the presence of red spots in the centre of which white pustules are likely to be present. This type of psoriasis occurs in less than 5% of people with psoriasis and is usually only seen in adults.

Regardless of the particular type of psoriasis an individual suffers, it usually causes at least a degree of discomfort that in some cases can range from mild to severe pain. For psoriasis sufferers, it is a fact of their life that their skin itches almost always, and that it can often also crack and bleed.

In the most severe cases, the pain suffered by a person suffering from psoriasis may be significant enough to prevent them from carrying out daily tasks, while making established sleep extremely difficult.

In medical terms, the treatment that medical professionals and other physicians would recommend for psoriasis will depend largely on the severity of the condition suffered by the person seeking advice.

Some dermatologists would classify psoriasis into three different categories, being mild, moderate and severe with the definition of each of these categories depending on the percentage of the patient's body that is covered with psoriasis lesions.

By these standards, anyone who has lesions covering between 5% and 10% of their body would fall into the mild category, between 10% and 20% would be moderate, and anyone who has more than 20% of their body covered by psoriasis lesions would fall into the severe category.

It has already been suggested that up to 20% of the U.S. population (and by extension of the rest of the western world) can suffer psoriasis, and that the vast majority falls into the category of mild or even very mild. For many of these people, their condition is nothing more than mild discomfort with moderate skin lesions and minor itching, often temporarily.

At the other end of the scale, there are some unfortunates whose condition is so severe that they develop injuries all over the body and have to be hospitalized in order for the condition to be treated. For these people, their psoriasis is likely to be extremely painful and can also be disfiguring and even potentially disabling.

And unfortunately, because psoriasis is a chronic disease, meaning that it is a life-long illness, there can be no total relief for anyone who suffers from it. Psoriasis is a disease that can apparently disappear and reappear (often with a vengeance) many times throughout life, and as there is no recognised cure for the disease, it is a fact that everyone who suffers from psoriasis has to get used to and live with.

Causes of psoriasis

As in the case of a surprising number of medical conditions, the exact causes of psoriasis have yet to be established beyond doubt. But, while the traditional view of psoriasis was that it is a condition of the epidermis, the highest layer of skin, research in recent years has begun to indicate the opposite.

This research has indicated that far from being a condition that is only related to the epidermis, the causes of psoriasis are much deeper. In fact, this research indicates that psoriasis is a disease caused by malfunctioning of the patient's immune system when certain immune cells are activated and then become hyperactive.

In any individual who has a perfectly functioning immune system, white blood cells or T-cells produce antibodies that are designed to repel bacteria and viruses. However, it is now believed that in the case of a person with psoriasis, these cells begin to fight an imaginary infection or try to heal a wound that does not exist by creating an excess of new skin cells to repel the imaginary invader or to repair non-existent damage.

This in turn leads to the appearance of plaques or skin lesions that are endemic to plaque psoriasis.

Under normal circumstances, the life cycle of an average skin cell for someone who is totally healthy is about 28 days, but it is believed that in people with psoriasis, their immune system is creating too many cells. In addition, because these cells are being produced so quickly, they mature in just three to six days before moving to the surface of the skin.

Consequently, because these cells are not dying fast enough, they accumulate on the surface of the skin, layer upon layer, and thus psoriatic plaques form.

Thanks to this research, we now have what is believed to be a reasonably accurate idea of what causes psoriasis.

What we do not know, however, is exactly why some individuals suffer from psoriasis and others do not.

On the other hand, there are some generally accepted factors that make some individuals more prone to psoriasis than others.

> ## *Why do people have psoriasis?*

Research indicates that around 30% of people who develop psoriasis have a family history of the disease, but it is also true that many parents who suffer from psoriasis will have children who do not have problems of their own. On the other hand, there will be people who develop psoriasis who do not have a family history of the disease, so suggesting that psoriasis is hereditary might be a little misleading.

However, it is true that researchers have established that there are certain genetic combinations and/or mutations that seem to predispose anyone who has them to psoriasis.

Currently, researchers believe there are nine different genetic mutations that could play a role in making certain people predisposed to psoriasis. However, there is a particular mutation of chromosome 6 known as PSORS-1 (for susceptibility to psoriasis 1) that appears to be the particular mutation that plays the most important role in deciding who is likely to have psoriasis and who is not.

According to a study published in the American Journal of Human Genetics in 2006, research has established that the role of this particular genetic mutation was observed in more than 2,700 psoriasis sufferers from nearly 680 families in which one or both parents suffered from psoriasis.

Today, the scientific and research community agrees that this particular mutation causes T cells to behave differently, hence the connection to psoriasis.

But it is also the fact that this particular genetic mutation does not necessarily mean that an individual is certain of psoriasis. In fact, the same research study by James T. Elder, MD, PhD, suggests that for every individual with the PSORS-1 gene that develops psoriasis, there will be 10 other individuals carrying exactly the same gene who do not develop the disease.

On the other hand, it should also be noted that many of the same mutations thought to predispose a person to psoriasis may also have a connection to other immune-mediated conditions, such as type 1 diabetes or rheumatoid arthritis.

Therefore, although some people who have a particular genetic mutation may be more prone to psoriasis, it is possible that instead of having psoriasis, they may have diabetes or rheumatoid arthritis.

In fact, while the risk of developing psoriasis increases if one or both parents also suffer, the risks of developing other immune-mediated conditions, especially Crohn's disease or diabetes, increase in the same situation.

From all this, it might be natural to assume that having some family history of psoriasis probably means that you will develop psoriasis yourself, but in many cases, this simply doesn't happen.

Therefore, we should ask ourselves, why (or not) does this happen?

Why do people suffer from psoriasis?

Since there are some people whose genetic makeup predisposes them to psoriasis, why don't all people with this particular genetic makeup suffer? Alternatively, why is it that some people with exactly the same genetic make-up "psoriasis-friendly" end up with type 1 diabetes instead of psoriasis?

The answer seems to be that there has to be some kind of trigger for the immune system of a person with psoriasis to start creating skin cells at such an accelerated rate that they suffer an outbreak of skin lesions.

Many different forms of triggers have been reported and suggested, such as:

- Skin abrasions, cuts, and other injuries;
- increased emotional stress or anxiety
- Cold, humid or cloudy weather;
- Strep or other infections, including something as basic and simple as a sore throat;
- Sunburn.

In addition, it is also believed that certain medications can cause psoriasis, especially in those already genetically predisposed to the disease.

This category includes a wide variety of medications ranging from common or garden medications, everyday home remedies such as aspirin to beta-blockers (medications used to fight high blood pressure and certain heart conditions), antimalarial medications, and lithium.

Dermatologists have reported that they have seen psoriasis develop suddenly in people who have not previously had any skin problems or lesions in a very short period of time after starting one of these medications or after they have had (for example) a sore throat or sunburn.

In essence, while it appears that people who already have a genetic predisposition to psoriasis are more likely to develop the disease than others who do not, each individual appears to be different.

Although almost everyone with psoriasis saw their condition begin due to some kind of trigger, not everyone falls into the same category.

For a relatively small number of people, psoriasis almost seems to appear out of nowhere, probably because there was some trigger in their life (for example, a relatively minor but nevertheless stressful event at that time) that they have long forgotten.

What triggers psoriasis varies and differs from individual to individual. In addition, even a combination of PSORS-1 and a trigger or even several triggers does not necessarily mean that psoriasis is the inevitable result.

> ### *The development of psoriasis*

As a general observation, psoriasis first develops in relatively young people, often in adolescence or early adulthood. However, it is not unknown that psoriasis manifests itself in much younger children, nor is it impossible for it to develop later in life.

And as previously suggested, because psoriasis is a chronic disease, it's something you carry with you for the rest of your life.

However, this does not mean for a moment that psoriasis is a constant. In fact, for most patients, it is a condition that will vary in severity throughout their lives depending on lifestyle factors at any given time.

For example, it is very common for someone who has psoriasis to suffer the most severe outbreaks at times of greatest stress, while the opposite is also true, so that their visible psoriasis almost disappears at times when they are most relaxed.

The same is true when you have an infection that can trigger an attack, while sometimes, when infections are not a problem, the severity of psoriasis is likely to decrease.

When you understand the connection between your immune system and the prevalence of psoriasis, this notion of being "attacked" at its lowest point makes a lot of sense.

At that point, your immune system is at its weakest - when you are anxious or stressed - or alternatively at its strongest, working overtime to produce T-cells to fight infections or heal wounds. In both cases, the crucial factor is that your immune system is unbalanced and therefore your T-cell count is also out of control, hence vulnerability to an outbreak of more serious injuries.

Quality of life and psoriasis

As noted above, there are five different types of psoriasis, all of which vary in severity from mild to severe. However, regardless of the particular type of psoriasis you suffer from or the degree of severity, it is a fact that anyone or all psoriasis sufferers may find that their quality of life is adversely affected by their disease.

For many people, even those suffering from very mild psoriasis, anxiety, stress, loneliness, low self-esteem and lack of confidence are constant factors in their daily lives. As there is little difference between the prevalence of psoriasis in men and women, it is very easy for sufferers of both sexes to feel that their condition makes them unattractive and unpopular.

Since most people develop psoriasis in their teens and early 20s, it is especially cruel that the condition tends to develop at a time when most people want to be more attractive to the opposite sex. Consequently, although it is entirely possible that the condition is not physically harmful in any way, it is perfectly feasible that it can be extremely harmful in a psychological way.

This is confirmed by a study that suggested that suicidal thoughts are three times more common in people with psoriasis than in a directly comparable control group of people who do not suffer from the disease.

Another extremely common emotional reaction that most psoriasis sufferers will recognize is shame. To put it bluntly, it's simply not pleasant if you recognize that you have scaly skin and that other people feel uncomfortable or even repelled by your condition.

For example, many psoriasis sufferers also suffer from psoriasis on the scalp, which means that most people probably assume that you have extraordinarily bad dandruff. This is bad enough in everyday life, but it gets considerably worse if you need to go to the hairdresser.

And, although psoriasis is not contagious and, therefore, it is not possible for anyone else to "catch" it from a person who has it, the rest of the world who does not suffer from psoriasis is not always aware of this fact. As a result, most people with psoriasis report situations in which others seemed to hesitate to shake hands or otherwise make skin-to-skin contact.

In addition, studies have indicated that people who suffer from psoriasis often find that life becomes increasingly frustrating as a result of their illness. This is because psoriasis often limits their ability to do the things they did before the condition began, sometimes making it difficult or even impossible to perform the basic tasks required as part of their normal work routine.

As a result, the National Psoriasis Foundation has reported that people with psoriasis lose up to 56 million hours of work each year as a result of their illness. In addition, the same organization reported that more than a quarter of people with psoriasis had found it necessary to interrupt or change their normal daily activities as a result of psoriasis in a study conducted in 2002.

In addition to all these psychological and emotional factors, there are, of course, many physical disadvantages to having psoriasis.

Itching to a greater or lesser degree is common for almost everyone with psoriasis, and cracked, bleeding skin is also extremely common. For many people with psoriasis, pain is a daily constant and some aspects of having the condition, such as psoriasis on the nails, can be very painful.

Medical treatments for psoriasis

As mentioned above, there is currently no recognized cure for psoriasis.

However, there are many different forms of treatment that will be more or less effective depending on the specific type of psoriasis you have and the severity of your condition. Therefore, there is no form of treatment that is used or recommended as a "comprehensive" medical treatment for psoriasis.

Now, before you move on to the treatment stage, the first thing you should do is establish that the skin condition you have is, in fact, one form of psoriasis or another. This is not possible on your own, so you will need to consult a dermatologist or other recognized physician for a professional diagnosis of your condition.

Once the condition of which you have been confirmed as psoriasis, it is likely that the dermatologist will recommend a particular type of treatment, the selection depending on a number of factors such as:

✓ The specific type of psoriasis you have been diagnosed with;

✓ The severity of the condition, often measured by the percentage of skin affected;

✓ Your age, medical history, and general health;

✓ The location of the psoriatic lesions and

✓ The general effects that your condition seems to be having on you in terms of your physical and emotional well-being.

Once the answers to all of these questions have been established, your dermatologist will be able to recommend a particular type of treatment. And again, these treatment methods can be divided into several different categories:

✓ If your psoriasis is mild to moderate, topical treatments, creams, or lotions that may be applied to the affected area may be recommended;

✓ Systematic treatments, those taken by mouth or injected may be the recommended option if psoriasis is more severe or if

✓ In some cases, phototherapy (i.e., treatment by applying light to affected areas) or laser therapy may be recommended.

Let's consider each of these different types of treatment to consider how they work, how effective they can be, and whether there are hazards or potential side effects that you may need to be aware of.

> *Topical treatments for psoriasis*

There are several different types of

topical treatments for psoriasis, some of which are potentially more dangerous than others. The main treatments you may find or recommend to buy from your dermatologist or other medical professional are as follows.

Anthralin: Anthralin is a synthetic substitute for a natural substance known as chrysarobine that was originally extracted from the bark of the araroba tree that is the most common in South America.

The original natural substance was used to treat psoriasis for at least 100 years, and both the original substance and the synthetic substitute proved very effective in treating the plaques commonly associated with psoriasis vulgaris.

Antraline is believed to act on psoriatic lesions by normalizing the growth rate of skin cells, gradually reducing the accumulation of individual plaque areas to minimize inflammation.

Although antraline is not as effective as topical steroids, it also does not have the known long-term side effects. However, it can cause skin irritation, and it is not uncommon for anthralin to leave permanent stains on almost everything it touches, including clothing and even bathroom furniture.

Coal tar cream or ointment: As the name most likely suggests, coal tar is a thick lignite that is extracted as a by-product of coal carbonization. It is a product that has a strong odor that many people find unpleasant or unpleasant, but it is also one of the oldest known treatments for psoriasis, and in many situations, it is very effective in treating moderate to mild psoriasis.

There are many different preparations for psoriasis with coal tar, some of which can be purchased without a prescription at the local pharmacy. These different formulations are used to treat inflammation, flaking and itching, and can come in creams that are applied directly to the affected area, shampoo (coal tar is effective for psoriasis of the scalp) and even in a solution that is added to bath water that apparently helps delay the development of new lesions.

The main advantage of coal tar as a treatment for psoriasis is that, since the base materials are cheap and abundant, the treatment itself is usually not expensive. On the other hand, many people find the smell of coal tar repugnant, and because of the dark coloration, it tends to stain everything it touches.

In addition, some people with psoriasis find that using coal tar over a long period of time can cause unpleasant skin irritation, which is the last thing anyone with a naturally itchy condition needs.

Tazarotene: Tazarotene is a man-made derivative of vitamin A that is commonly prescribed for different types of skin conditions, including psoriasis, sunburn, and acne. It is generally used to treat mild to moderate psoriasis vulgaris, while it has also been used to treat psoriasis on nails with some degree of success.

Tazarotene commonly causes local skin irritation when applied, and is known to be most effective when used in conjunction with topical corticosteroids.

It works by normalizing skin cell production activity and is known to be effective in more difficult-to-treat areas of the body, such as knees and elbows.

However, in addition to known skin irritation, other similar vitamin A derivatives are known to have been implicated in causing birth defects when taken systematically. Although topical application of a substance of this type is much less dangerous than systematic ingestion, it is true that the use of tazarotene during pregnancy may not be too prudent.

Corticosteroids: The most potent and effective topical treatments for psoriasis are undoubtedly corticosteroids, but they are also the treatment that carries the greatest risk of long-term adverse side effects. However, due to their effectiveness in reducing inflammation and itching while slowing the rate of skin cell growth, corticosteroids are probably the most commonly prescribed topical treatment for psoriasis.

Corticosteroid treatments come in several different concentrations ranging from relatively mild to extremely strong, but prolonged use of these substances could have noticeable adverse side effects. For example, corticosteroids are recognized to cause thinning of the skin, excess body hair, dilate blood vessels, and can lead to infections that invade the body as well (often due to thinned skin).

In addition, it is believed that they can inhibit growth in children and that long-term use makes them increasingly ineffective, without preventing adverse side effects.

The bottom line is that the use of corticosteroid creams, potions or lotions to treat psoriasis could result in many more problems than they solve, and therefore it is something you want to avoid doing if possible.

➢ *Systematic treatments for psoriasis*

For moderate to mild psoriasis, topical treatments are usually the first solution a dermatologist or doctor will recommend. However, in a situation where the condition is considered more serious, they are probably more likely to recommend some form of routine treatment.

Since routine treatments are often prescribed only for severe and severe psoriasis, it follows that the drugs used are considerably more potent. As a result, possible side effects are also much more dangerous.

Acitretin: Acitretin is a powerful vitamin A derivative (a retinoid) taken orally under medical supervision. This particular systematic treatment has been shown to be effective in treating both erythrodermic and pustular psoriasis and works particularly well when used in combination with phototherapy.

However, side effects can be very unpleasant or dangerous, so constant medical attention and supervision is absolutely necessary. Possible side effects include severe headaches, increased blood lipid levels, hair loss, dry or clammy skin, and joint pain.

Cyclosporine: Cyclosporine is a very potent immunosuppressive drug that is effective in treating severe plaque psoriasis and nail psoriasis. Although it is a very potent and effective treatment, it is generally reserved for those patients for whom other forms of psoriasis treatment have not worked due to the possibility of serious adverse side effects, including irreparable kidney damage.

Methotrexate: Methotrexate was one of the first commonly used chemotherapeutic drugs still used to treat moderate to severe psoriasis. Although extremely effective, this is another systematic treatment that needs to be carefully monitored because of the possibility of serious and lasting liver damage.

As you have probably already realised, all of the routine psoriasis treatments that are commonly used to treat moderate to moderate psoriasis are very potent medicines. It is therefore not surprising that all of them have potentially serious side effects and can only be used under strict medical supervision.

Given the obvious danger inherent in taking systematic psoriasis treatments such as these, it obviously makes sense to seek natural alternatives whenever possible.

➢ *Phototherapy and laser treatment for psoriasis*

Some of the treatments already mentioned (e.g. acetritin) work even more effectively when combined with phototherapy, which is usually the application of ultraviolet light or the use of a laser.

As for the use of ultraviolet light to treat psoriasis, it is possible to undergo treatment with ultraviolet A light or ultraviolet B light, and although the two work very similarly, there are some differences.

In both cases, ultraviolet light is applied to the area of the injury over a period of time, and in both cases, the treatment is highly effective. However, on the negative side, both forms of UV treatment require many visits to the clinic or hospital over a period of time, and also have their negative side.

In the case of UVA treatment, there is

an increased risk of skin freckles, aging, and even skin cancer in a case where a patient has suffered prolonged exposure to UVA light. In addition, side effects may include nausea, headaches, burning or itching of the skin, irregular skin pigmentation, and general fatigue.

When it comes to UVB treatment, it is more likely that the patient will have to undergo other treatments, since although phototherapy is effective in eliminating lesions, it tends to do so less permanently. And, once again, long-term exposure to UVB light increases the risk of skin cancer.

On the other hand, laser therapy is much more powerful than any of the ultraviolet light treatments, but at the same time, it is also much more targeted. This is an advantage of a way in which the use of laser light to reduce or eliminate injuries is extremely effective, but it also means that only a relatively small area of the body can be treated at any given time.

In addition, the treatment can sometimes be painful, while it can also cause irregular darkening of the skin and scarring.

Again, although phototherapy and laser treatment are very effective, both have significant disadvantages. Therefore, you should consider the natural solutions that I will propose in the next two chapters before undergoing potentially harmful drugs or pharmaceutical treatments that could cause complications.

However, you should also understand that there may be situations where your psoriasis cannot be treated with all-natural methods, mainly because natural treatments are almost always much milder and less invasive than the stronger chemical-based pharmaceuticals.

However, unless your psoriasis is classified as severe or severe, it makes sense to consider the use of natural forms of treatment before considering the use of potent chemicals in or on your body.

Only after experimenting with natural solutions and discovering that they can do nothing for you, should you turn to the chemical medications that your physician assistant or dermatologist will certainly recommend.

The best natural treatments

As medical science has not yet succeeded in finding a cure for psoriasis, it should be obvious that nature, unfortunately, has also not been able to provide a complete cure.

However, there are many different natural treatments that you can prove to be effective for different people at different times in alleviating, reducing or eliminating the plaques and lesions that are the most common external indication of psoriasis.

Unfortunately, it is almost impossible to know exactly what is going to be effective for a particular individual, so to a large extent, finding what works for you is likely to be a trial and error process. That said, there are many options you can try to see if they alleviate or calm your condition, so all of the following alternatives are worthy of consideration.

➢ *Acupuncture for psoriasis*

Based on the medical practices of ancient China, acupuncture is a system for treating pain and disease by applying needles to certain parts of the body. However, these needles are generally not inserted into the body at the point where the complaint or problem is most evident, because the thought behind acupuncture is that the body contains a network of "roads" along which signals travel.

Therefore, it is more common for acupuncture needles to be inserted into the "road" at a point on the body far away from the place of complaint as a way of diverting signals to places they are supposed to go, or away from places where they are not.

However, although acupuncture has been used for many centuries to treat a wide range of ailments and medical conditions, it has never been recognized as a treatment for psoriasis in China, mainly because in most Asian countries, psoriasis is an extremely rare disease (on the other hand, it is more common in Scandinavia).

However, Western practitioners of acupuncture believe that acupuncture can be a very effective treatment for psoriasis, although there is little clinical evidence to support these claims and what is effective in treating one person's psoriasis will vary greatly from what works best for another person.

Although it may take a few sessions of acupuncture before you see positive and visible results, the "advantage" of treating a condition with acupuncture is that there are no possible side effects. In addition, even if you are afraid of needles, there are many acupuncturists who now use the application of electric currents using probes instead of needles that are probably as effective as the traditional acupuncturist who wields the needles.

> ## ➢ *You are what you eat*

Although the headline may be a bit of a cliché, it is never less true that each and every human being on the face of the Earth is made up of everything they have eaten or drunk in their lifetime. Therefore, it follows that just as psoriasis is an integral part of you, so is your diet. Therefore, it is not absurd to assume that one has some effect on the other.

Trying to eat a diet that helps keep psoriasis under control is about maintaining a well-balanced diet that contributes to overall well-being, while avoiding foods that could exacerbate the situation.

For example, according to the prestigious dermatologist Janet Prystowsky, there are many studies that support the idea that psoriasis has a tendency to cause certain nutritional deficiencies in people who suffer from it.

Therefore, anyone with psoriasis should focus on replacing these missing nutrients by adding extra protein and folate (from green leafy vegetables) to their diet. In addition, drinking more water and iron will not necessarily help eliminate psoriasis, but it will improve your overall well-being, which is important, because the stronger you are, the less likely you are to experience outbreaks of psoriatic lesions.

Although this is probably not a surprise, many studies have indicated that a balanced, low-fat diet can help prevent many serious medical conditions such as strokes, heart disease, and cancer. What is perhaps less well known is that some doctors have noticed that the skin of psoriasis sufferers often improves when they follow a well-controlled diet to lose weight, while those who are gaining weight will probably see an increase in psoriasis outbreaks.

Again, there is a lot of common sense in this, because we have already established that stress and anxiety can increase outbreaks of psoriasis, while the opposite is also true. Working on the assumption that someone who is on a well-controlled diet to lose weight is voluntarily losing weight, it naturally follows that they are happier since they are losing weight, which could have some bearing on their improved condition.

The National Psoriasis Foundation suggests that they have received many reports from members indicating that eliminating or at least reducing certain foods in their diet has led to significant skin improvements. Foods or ingredients to avoid include caffeine, alcohol, white flour, purified sugar, and all gluten-containing products.

Other tips for a diet that does not encourage psoriasis flare include:

✓ Eat only easily digestible foods and avoid overly spicy foods;

✓ Don't include too many salty, acidic, or sour foods in your diet;

✓ Including more fruits and vegetables in the diet is always good for overall health, but bitter squash, steamed vegetables, and pumpkin are thought to be particularly good for a "psoriasis-friendly" diet;

✓ Avoid too much animal fat and eggs;

✓ Include plenty of fatty fish rich in omega-3 fatty acids, or take supplements of cod liver oil, lecithin, or flaxseed oil.

Other natural treatments for psoriasis

Oats: It's no coincidence that there are so many skin care products on the market that use oats as one of their main components, because oat extract has been used for many centuries as a topical soothing agent to control and soothe itchy or irritated skin. There are many ways to use oatmeal to take advantage of its calming and calming qualities:

✓ Drink 1 cup dry oatmeal and 1/4 cup dry milk before mixing in 2 tablespoons apricot kernel oil. Slowly grind the mixture in a food blender before putting it in a muslin bag or, failing that, in an old sock. Drop the bag or sock in a hot bath and then gently squeeze the water from the contents of the bag into the affected areas of your skin, as this releases the beneficial ingredients of the mixture to soothe your skin.

✓ Look for body lotions and moisturizers that use oats or oat extract as their main active ingredient. Apply the moisturizing cream abundantly in the morning and evening, focusing especially on the affected areas of the skin.

✓ Make an oatmeal pad by wrapping the oatmeal in a cloth

bag, soaking it in buttermilk, and applying the pad to any affected area of your skin. This combines two materials (oats and curd) that are both believed to have healing effects, so you should expect to see the results of this particular method fairly quickly.

Aloe: There are approximately 500 different species of aloe currently known, but the most commonly used and best-known is aloe. Secretion from the leaves of this particular plant has long been used as a treatment for burns and minor skin damage, but in 1996, a study published in the journal Tropical Medicine and International Health suggested for the first time that aloe vera might also be very effective in the treatment of psoriasis.

During this study, conducted over a period of 16 weeks, it was established that the use of a cream containing aloe vera indicated a significant clearance of psoriasis lesions in 25 out of 30 test individuals, compared to only 2 individuals in the control group. On the other hand, it has to be said that a more recent study suggests that the use of commercial aloe vera may not be as effective as suggested, but since there is no likelihood of adverse side effects from applying aloe vera to your plaques, it is definitely something worth trying as a topical treatment for psoriasis and psoriatic arthritis.

An alternative or additional way to use aloe vera to help in the fight against psoriasis is to drink the juice of the plant. Although some proponents of aloe vera recommend growing your own plants from which you can expect this juice, they are notoriously difficult to grow successfully, so it's probably best to buy juice prepared for drinking.

The benefits of doing so are widespread, and many of them are directly applicable to people with psoriasis or psoriatic arthritis. For example, for the person suffering from arthritis, aloe vera is known to contain 12 all-natural substances that have been shown to counteract inflammation without any adverse side effects.

In addition, aloe vera juice contains many vital vitamins and nutrients that will contribute to your overall well-being, plus it has the ability to help your skin regenerate and repair itself in the shortest time possible.

Apple Cider Vinegar: Again, according to the National Psoriasis Foundation, many individual members report that the use of apple cider vinegar has led to significant improvements in their psoriasis. These members suggest adding vinegar to your bath, applying it directly to psoriatic nails, and even applying it directly to affected areas of the skin using balls or cotton buds.

Alternatively, you can try to attack your psoriasis and/or psoriatic arthritis internally by adding apple cider vinegar to your diet. While many people would find that drinking pure apple cider vinegar is difficult - it is very acidic or bitter - it can be added to warm water with honey to sweeten the potion before drinking it. Do this at least twice a day, and you will be attacking your psoriasis-related problem from the inside in the most effective way possible.

The effectiveness of apple cider vinegar should not be particularly surprising because vinegar has been used throughout history as a curative solution, and the medicinal benefits of apple cider vinegar have long been well known.

Capsaicin: Derived from cayenne peppers, capsaicin when applied to the skin has been shown in some studies to reduce redness, minimize flaking and also eliminate itching. This is thought to happen because capsaicin disrupts the activity of a molecule that affects the way the brain recognizes itching and pain known as substance P.

It is for this reason that many over-the-counter arthritis pain relief products contain capsaicin, and certainly in several trials with different groups of people suffering from psoriasis, a topical application of 0.025% cream on affected skin areas definitely reduced desquamation, redness and itching.

On the negative side, some individuals reported a short-lived burning sensation, but if you are willing to risk this happening to you, then applying a very weak capsaicin solution to your injuries could bring you much sought-after relief.

Tea Tree Oil: Tea tree oil is extracted from the Melaleuca Alternifolia tree which is native to Australia, and has been used in surgery and dentistry for nearly 100 years. Tea tree oil is widely known for its antiseptic and antibacterial qualities, and has traditionally been used for headaches, toothaches, colds, rheumatisms, muscle aches and skin conditions.

However, it would be very unwise to treat toothache with tea tree oil because it is toxic if ingested. In addition, it has not been established at what level or concentration of tea tree oil is most effective, so if you decide to use it, you should do so with some degree of caution.

Tea tree oil is not only disinfectant and soothing, it also has the ability to penetrate deep beneath the skin, well below the upper epidermal level. This is especially important for a person with psoriasis, because it means that the antifungal, disinfectant and healing qualities of the oil penetrate deep into the skin, helping to regulate the production of psoriatic plaques in the early stages.

Although it is extremely unlikely that you will suffer any real damage from tea tree oil, you should desist from using it if you feel any discomfort in your skin.

Milk Thistle: Milk thistle has been

shown to inhibit the production of T cells, so although no specific testing has been done on the efficacy of milk thistle as a treatment for psoriasis, the fact that it can stop the growth of the cells that cause it suggests it is worth a try. You can buy milk thistle products at the health store or pharmacy in liquid or tablet form, and there are no adverse side effects other than minor gastrointestinal disorders when you start taking the supplement for the first time.

Oregano Oil: Oregano is a spice commonly used in cooking that has antibacterial and antifungal qualities that may be helpful in keeping at bay some of the infections that may be associated with psoriasis. Oregano can be safely ingested in almost any form, and many people report that taking a daily 'dose' of oregano has significantly helped keep their psoriasis under control.

Turmeric: Turmeric is a popular ingredient in Indian curry, and although you can buy this spice back as a food supplement, it is easier and much cheaper to mix the spice into your meal (no more than one teaspoon is needed). Turmeric has been shown to help reduce inflammation in all parts of the body, including the skin, as well as relieve the pain and swelling associated with arthritis.

Shark Cartilage: Studies conducted in recent years indicate that shark cartilage extract may help delay the formation of new blood and skin cells, which are both believed to play an important role in the development and growth of psoriatic lesions. Shark cartilage is also believed to have highly effective anti-inflammatory qualities.

A particular form of shark cartilage AE-941 (known by the brand name Neovastat) has shown great promise as a treatment for psoriasis, but it is not yet widely approved for general use, because the long-term effects of its use are unknown and, in the short term, it has

been observed to cause nausea and
vomiting.

Psoriatic arthritis

Another complication suffered by up to 30% of people with psoriasis is a condition known as psoriatic arthritis.

Regardless of the particular type of psoriasis you have or the degree of severity of the condition, it is still possible to develop psoriatic arthritis, which is a life-long condition that causes pain and stiffness in the joint, accompanied by gradual deterioration.

The signs that you may be developing psoriatic arthritis are:

    ✓ Red, inflamed psoriatic skin lesions around the joint area;

    ✓ Pain and swelling in the joints that is worse in the morning or after a rest period;

    ✓ fingernail and toenail irregularities, such as nails that

begin to fall off nail beds, stings, orange or yellow discoloration, or unusual ridge patterns

Psoriatic arthritis is most often seen in the joints of the fingers and toes, but other critical bone joints such as the knees, elbows, ankles, and neck may also be affected in some individuals. No matter what joints are affected, the area around the joint is almost always stiff and painful, and often tends to have a darker color. You may also notice that the affected area feels warmer to the touch than the unaffected surrounding areas.

Psoriatic arthritis can vary in severity and symptoms from person to person. For example, while some people will suffer "completely" psoriatic arthritis, others will suffer only mild joint stiffness.

In addition, despite the name of the condition, not only people who already have psoriasis develop psoriatic arthritis.

However, about 70% of people who

develop the disease already have psoriasis. In this situation, studies indicate that in most people, arthritis will begin about 10 years after first suffering psoriasis, although cases have been reported in which arthritis begins within months of the initial diagnosis of psoriasis.

As a general guideline, most people with psoriatic arthritis will probably see the first signs of the condition between the ages of 30 and 50.

As with all forms of arthritis, psoriatic arthritis can be a debilitating and paralyzing condition, but unfortunately, it is extremely easy to confuse the first warning signs of the condition with dozens of other possibilities. For example, it is generally recognized that common early warning signs include lateral elbow pain (generally known as "tennis elbow") or pain in the hands or feet.

Obviously, it is extremely easy to conclude that such things can happen to anyone for any reason and simply ignore them, especially if there are no recognizable plaques visible or evident. Similarly, pain in the shoulder, neck, or upper back may be the first signs of psoriatic arthritis, but again, these warning signs would be extremely easy to confuse and, as a result, "just one of those things" could be ignored.

However, once psoriatic arthritis begins to appear, about 9 out of 10 people who suffer will begin to see the disease manifest through the fingernails and toenails. In this case, the affected person may begin to see that their nails begin to move away from the nail bed or that bite marks and discoloration become evident.

As soon as these physiological changes occur, it is very important that anyone suffering from psoriasis consult their doctor immediately, as it is possible to stop the deterioration of joints with proper treatment.

And of course, there are natural treatments you can use to compensate for the worst effects of psoriatic arthritis, but we'll come back to them a little later.

It may not be surprising that psoriatic arthritis and its effects vary in severity from individual to individual. However, the effects of psoriatic arthritis can be extremely serious.

For example, according to statistics from the National Psoriasis Foundation, approximately one in five people with psoriatic arthritis has damage to five or more joints in their body, which means that their quality of life and their ability to perform the basic tasks of daily living are severely impaired.

And then, of course, there are people at the opposite end of the spectrum who suffer only slight stiffness in the joints. However, even for these people, it must be accepted that the condition can always get worse.

➢ *Causes of psoriatic arthritis*

Even in people who get psoriatic arthritis and who did not previously suffer from psoriasis, it is generally believed that the main cause of psoriatic arthritis is remarkably similar to that of psoriasis.

For example, it seems likely that psoriatic arthritis is caused by a defect in the patient's immune system. In addition, it seems likely that people with psoriatic arthritis are often genetically predisposed to do so and need some kind of psychological, emotional or physical trigger to trigger the onset of arthritis in exactly the same way as with psoriasis.

➢ *Who can suffer from psoriatic arthritis?*

In the U.S. it is believed that there are about one million people who suffer from psoriatic arthritis, and most of the people who have suffered from it before, particularly pustular psoriasis.

Most commonly, the effect of psoriatic arthritis is felt by people who already suffer from psoriasis and who are between 30 and 50 years of age. However, it is not unknown that even young children develop psoriatic arthritis.

Girls between the ages of 2 and 4 are known to suffer from psoriatic arthritis, and the best time for the disease to catch on in boys between the ages of 11 and 12 is for both boys and girls. The most worrying thing is that it is even known that arthritis starts even before psoriasis has appeared, although because it is extremely rare, this would not necessarily be something that most parents without a family history of psoriasis should be too concerned about.

> ### *Diagnosis and recognition of symptoms of psoriatic arthritis*

The number one goal for anyone who suspects they may be susceptible to psoriatic arthritis is to know how to recognize the onset of the condition as early as possible.

Of course, the condition is not called psoriatic arthritis in vain. Most people who suffer are those who have previously suffered psoriasis, so that would be the first clue that they are susceptible to the disease.

Second, any unexplained pain, particularly around the joints, may be giving you a clue that psoriatic arthritis is a "target" for you. Most sick people are within a certain age range (30-50), so this is where you are?

It is important to understand that once psoriatic arthritis begins to appear, the deterioration of the joints and the corresponding increase in pain can begin to accelerate very quickly, so you must do something to stop this acceleration.

As most people who have found someone who suffers from arthritis probably understand, it is not a particularly difficult condition to recognize, but it is not easy to recognize the difference between the different types of arthritis if you are not medically qualified. After all, how many unqualified people could tell the difference between someone with rheumatoid arthritis or psoriatic arthritis?

The bottom line is that, if you do nothing about psoriatic arthritis, it is perfectly feasible that you will end up being able to do nothing about it because of your condition. Therefore, it is imperative that if you have any reason to suspect that you may have a problem, consult a dermatologist or other recognized medical professional as soon as possible.

Medical treatments for psoriatic arthritis

The goals of psoriatic arthritis treatment can be divided into three different categories. These are the ones:

- ✓ To control symptoms first;
- ✓ In addition to inhibiting and controlling joint damage and deformities, and finally
- ✓ To prevent disability.

However, every person with psoriatic arthritis is different and, therefore, there is no single medical treatment that solves everyone's problems. For this reason, there are many different specific formulations of different medications used to treat people with psoriatic arthritis, but most of these medications fall under one of two categories.

Therefore, rather than dealing with each individual drug, it makes more sense to examine the two different classes of drugs to explain why they work and the possible adverse side effects of each.

Nonsteroidal anti-inflammatory drugs (NSAIDs): NSAIDs are drugs that help relieve pain, relieve stiffness in joints, and reduce the swelling too often associated with any form of arthritis. These particular medications are very commonly used by those who suffer from non-psoriatic arthritis, and may include home medications as common as aspirin and ibuprofen.

Obviously, the possible side effects of the particular NSAID you are taking will vary from drug to drug, but may include nausea, headaches, vomiting, diarrhea, lack of appetite, and dizziness. They may also stimulate water retention, which in turn may promote edema, and in the worst case, may cause kidney or liver failure, ulcers, and prolonged internal bleeding, especially after surgery.

Disease-modifying anti-rheumatic drugs (DMARDs): The use of DMARDs is generally considered to be a less effective way to treat psoriatic arthritis because, although they slow the development of the condition, they very rarely stop it or reverse it completely. In addition, because in many cases it takes six to eight months for the drug in question to have any positive effect, they are also generally considered to be slow-acting drugs.

Although it is not fully understood how DMARDs work, it is generally agreed that they produce a slowdown in the progression of psoriatic arthritis by slowing or otherwise modifying the activities of the patient's immune system.

However, again, depending on the particular type of medication you are prescribed, you need to be aware that there is a possibility of unpleasant and dangerous side effects.

These include stomach pain, diarrhea or constipation, nausea, vomiting, headache, and possibly a violent rash. In addition, there are potentially more dangerous side effects such as increased blood pressure, decreased white blood cell count (which may partly explain why they are effective in treating a psoriasis-related condition), hair loss and increased susceptibility to infection.

As with psoriasis itself, you can't help but conclude that, in some cases, the treatments that your dermatologist or physician's assistant might recommend may, in some cases, be as bad as if they were no worse than the medical condition for which they were prescribed.

Natural treatments for `soriatic arthritis

Perhaps it's not too surprising that many of the natural treatments you might use for psoriasis can also be effective in helping to deal with the swelling, stiffness, and joint pain associated with psoriatic arthritis as well.

For example, it is known that topically applied tea tree oil relieves muscle and joint pain, while adding turmeric to foods or taking it as a dietary supplement can help relieve inflammation and pain associated with any form of arthritis.

However, because psoriasis and psoriatic arthritis are two very different diseases, there are many other natural treatments that deserve your consideration if you suffer from psoriatic arthritis that may not be as applicable in the case of psoriasis.

Chondroitin and Glucosamine:
Chondroitin and glucosamine are natural sulfate solutions that you can use to reduce pain and slow the progression of osteoarthritis, which is the deterioration of cartilage between the joints of your bones. Both substances are found naturally in the body, and chondroitin is believed to improve water retention, which in turn maintains elasticity in cartilage between bones, while glucosamine promotes cartilage repair and production.

The National Psoriasis Foundation suggests that there are very few side effects with any of these substances and that your long-term safety history is well established. However, women who are pregnant or trying to get pregnant should not take them, and glucosamine is likely to increase blood sugar levels, so it is not recommended for diabetics.

Both can be found in tablet form in health stores, as can all of the following supplements.

S-Adenosyl Methionine (SAM-e):

SAM-e is a synthetic version of a chemical that is naturally manufactured by all animals. Helps produce and regulate hormones and neurotransmitters, which in turn regulate mood and emotions.

Most importantly for a psoriatic arthritis sufferer, SAM-e participates in the manufacture of glutathione that the liver uses as part of the body's toxin elimination process (toxins that can exacerbate both psoriasis and psoriatic arthritis), while helping to rebuild cartilage, which again reduces the pain and incidence of osteoarthritis.

Methylsulfonylmethane (MSM):

MSM, sometimes referred to as dimethylsulfone, is a natural chemical found in fruits, plants, and grains that is unfortunately destroyed by the body during food digestion.

To repair and maintain healthy joint and connective tissue functions, the body needs sulfur. Consequently, MSM is able to help people with psoriatic arthritis because it is a natural sulfate that supplements the often too low levels of sulfate that most people have. MSM have also been reported to have pain-relieving qualities and the ability to reduce inflammation, but there is little established evidence as to why this should be so.

It should also be noted that there is little scientific data on the long-term benefits or side effects of using MSM, so it should be used with some degree of caution.

> ***Herbs for treating psoriatic arthritis***

Nettles: Nettles are found almost everywhere, but they are nevertheless a true food supplement of nature. Including nettles in your diet can help reduce high blood pressure, minimize the worst effects of eczema, and relieve the pain and swelling associated with rheumatism.

Saffron: Saffron is a natural source of weak hydrochloric acid that helps remove uric acid from the body, which is beneficial because it is the uric acid that binds the extra calcium deposited in the bone joints with the bone itself. It also helps reduce lactic acid buildup.

Cassava extract: In tests conducted over the past two years, it has been suggested that the inclusion of cassava extract in their diet helped many people with arthritis to reduce the severity of their condition. Although cassava extract supplements can already be found in health food stores, tests are still underway. However, so far, the results seem extremely encouraging for anyone suffering from any form of arthritis or rheumatism.

Bogbean: Bogbean is an ancient remedy that has been shown to have important anti-inflammatory and tonic qualities, making it an ideal treatment for an arthritic condition.

Conclusion

As highlighted throughout this book, although there are many chemical drug-based treatments available for both psoriasis and psoriatic arthritis, there is also a wide range and a large number of natural treatments for these two conditions.

And as with almost any medical condition, because most natural treatments have few (if any) adverse side effects, it always makes sense to consider using a natural treatment method before using solutions based on chemical drugs that can treat the condition but cause other problems in the process of doing so.

For anyone suffering from psoriasis, it is an unfortunate fact that there is no known cure for the disease today. However, as you must understand by now, there are plenty of natural treatments that you can use to deal with your psoriasis or, in fact, with psoriatic arthritis that can reduce or even eliminate the worst effects of the condition.

Of course, you shouldn't totally ignore medical advice or recommendations, especially if your psoriasis or psoriatic arthritis is particularly severe. In some circumstances, there is no doubt that medical intervention is likely to be necessary to manage the worst cases of psoriasis and psoriatic arthritis, and if this is your case, you may need to consider medical advice.

However, in many cases, drug-based pharmaceuticals that can be used topically or systematically will automatically be recommended by your medical advisor, regardless of the severity of your psoriatic arthritis from psoriasis. In such circumstances, natural solutions may provide exactly the same amount of relief as pharmaceuticals. Therefore, once you know that psoriasis or psoriatic arthritis is your problem, it surely makes sense to try natural solutions before going back to pharmaceuticals.

Psoriasis is a condition that may be a plague in your life, but it doesn't have to be. Equally important, it is a condition that can be treated in a totally natural way.

Armed with the information you have read in this book, now is the time to start treating psoriasis in a completely natural way.

Now yes, I wish you the best in your results, and remember, everything is practical; theory without action is of no use to you.

A big hug, your friend, Jessy!

By the way, when you achieve your results little by little, I highly recommend you, if you want to learn how to do a complete natural detoxification, my book, on "HOW TO DO A COMPLETE NATURAL DEINTOXICATION", is a book that I am sure will help you a lot on your way to "good health".

Without further ado, you can find it in the Amazon search engine, like: "How to do a complete natural detox" or looking for my name, like: "Jessy M. Brown"... Once again I wish you success in your results!

www.ingramcontent.com/pod-product-compliance
Lightning Source LLC
Chambersburg PA
CBHW072108280526
45788CB00006B/2453